AFTER THE INVISIBLE BRAIN INJURY

WHAT IT IS AND DIFFERENT MODALITIES TO HEAL

Sheryl Gallo, PsyD &
Elaine Billy, BS, CHHT, OB

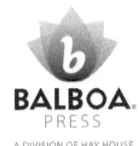

BALBOA.
PRESS

A DIVISION OF HAY HOUSE

Balboa Press books may be ordered through booksellers or by contacting:

Balboa Press
A Division of Hay House
1663 Liberty Drive
Bloomington, IN 47403
www.balboapress.com
1 (877) 407-4847

Because of the dynamic nature of the Internet, any web addresses or links contained in this book may have changed since publication and may no longer be valid. The views expressed in this work are solely those of the authors and do not necessarily reflect the views of the publisher, and the publisher hereby disclaims any responsibility for them.

There are certain parts and ideas in this book that we are uncertain of the source. It may be we heard it in a lecture, read it, had a class that covered it, saw it on television or received it in a meditation. None of the information was meant to be plagiarized. We have been using these theories and concepts in our practices for many years.

The authors of this book do not dispense medical advice or prescribe the use of any technique as a form of treatment for physical, emotional, or medical problems without the advice of a physician, either directly or indirectly. The intent of the authors is only to offer information of a general nature to help you in your quest for emotional and spiritual well-being. In the event you use any of the information in this book for yourself, which is your constitutional right, the authors and the publisher assume no responsibility for your actions.

Any people depicted in stock imagery provided by Thinkstock are models, and such images are being used for illustrative purposes only.
Certain stock imagery © Thinkstock.

Print information available on the last page.

ISBN: 978-1-5043-7086-8 (sc)
ISBN: 978-1-5043-7087-5 (e)

Library of Congress Control Number: 2016920057

Balboa Press rev. date: 10/22/2018

FOREWORD

The beginning of this book was written to describe the brain and its functioning. This may help you or your loved one who has suffered a brain injury understand the mechanism we call our brain.

The later portion of the book was written to give you hope and inspiration in dealing with injuries of any kind. We hope that the information we are including helps you and the injured party recover more quickly by providing the confidence and the knowledge to assist you in realizing you are not alone. We invite you to share the information.

CONTENTS

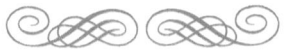

CHAPTER 1

Biology of the Brain

The brain is the main control system for our bodies. It seems that we take our brain for granted because we don't realize how much it controls our everyday functioning. The brain's physiological functioning is comparable to a fully stocked library. The brain has unique areas that categorize functioning. It archives a lot of information so that we retain the gathered information. The brain also has fuel to maintain its daily functioning, including the automatic nervous system which controls things like breathing, heart rate and automatic survival functions.

The brain consists of the following areas: frontal lobe, parietal lobe, temporal lobe, the occipital lobe, the cerebellum and the brain stem. The frontal lobe is responsible for our daily executive decisions, problem solving, planning, organizing, manipulating information, attention, focusing, sustaining attention and our abstract thinking (defined as those tasks we perform like math and puzzles). The parietal lobe regulates our senses such as our hearing, touch, vision, taste and smell. The temporal lobe manages memory including visual memory (remembering where we placed things), auditory memory (remembering what we just heard), semantic (the meaning of a word, phrase, sentence or text) and procedural or automatic memory (tasks such as remembering how to drive a car or ride a bicycle). The occipital lobe controls vision while the cerebellum regulates breathing, heart rate and internal regulation. The brain stem organizes everything as all the nerves travel through it. It all sounds simple and compartmentalized, however, the brain is much more complicated than what is stated, particularly when the brain becomes injured.

The physiological aspects of the brain are regulated by neurotransmitters. There are five major neurotransmitters which affect our emotions, thinking and behaviors on a daily basis. These neurotransmitters are: acetylcholine, norepinephrine, dopamine, serotonin and gamma aminobutyric acid. Acetylcholine helps with learning and memory. Norepinephrine plays an important role in regulating arousal and moods. Dopamine helps regulate motor movements of our bodies and helps us stay intact with reality. Serotonin regulates sleep and mood. Low serotonin levels have been implicated in depression. Finally, gamma aminobutyric keeps the brain from becoming too aroused or excited. Anxiety and some neurological disorders are linked to having low gamma aminobutyric.

It is amazing how our brains change biologically when learning and remembering information. This further supports the concept of neuroplasticity, how the brain re-wires and re-maps itself after injury or whenever necessary. This concept will be discussed in more detail in a later chapter. There is research that shows how DNA and RNA change as a result of learning new information. This is also an example of neuroplasticity. One particular theory is called cellular modification theory. This theory basically explains how the brain biologically re-wires itself when learning new information.

Most research that has supported the cellular modification theory has been through animal studies. Animal studies have contributed to our knowledge of biological and neurological changes that occur within the brain. There have been physiological studies of the hippocampus which indicate the synapses change and have lasting effects when learning and remembering information. Dated research on experimental rats teaching them to reach or not reach for food demonstrated that synaptic connections can be altered. The rats that were taught to reach for food had altered neuron changes in their motor cortex, suggesting synaptic changes associated with learning and memory (Fuch et al. 1983).

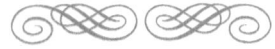

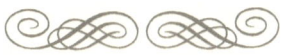

CHAPTER 2

The Brain Applied to Everyday Life

So, what do we need our brain for anyway? This is a simple question with a complicated answer. We need our brain for everything. It is our engine and our archival library. The easy answer is: it gets us going in the morning, it gets us to complete tasks, it makes us money, it makes us feel and think and so on. Without it we would be non-existent or just a body. From early childhood most parents or caretakers educate their young to take care of their bodies by eating healthy, exercising and getting plenty of restful sleep. Our society sends the messages to eat healthy and avoid illegal drugs in order to protect our brains. Unfortunately, when we injure our brain we want to do everything to speed up the healing. We are unsure of what to do or how to do it.

When the brain becomes injured, it turns one's world upside down. The injured person has limited understanding of how to get the brain back to normal. The problem with this is the lack of knowledge about healthy brain care and the lack of knowledge as to what the brain actually does. When the brain is injured, particularly the frontal lobe, it metabolizes differently compared to a non-injured brain. For example, the amygdala, which regulates emotional responses, regulates an on/off switch for eating. This on/off switch is regulated by dopamine. During brain injury this is thrown off, out of whack or places that on/off switch off kilter, thus creating difficulty in regulating eating. When this happens it deprives the brain of the important nutrients it needs. Therefore, it is important to consume the appropriate amounts of vitamins, minerals, water, proteins, fats and carbohydrates. For example, if you eat the right foods which increase the neurotransmitter serotonin in the brain, you will feel more relaxed. The same is true for consuming the foods that increase the dopamine and norepinephrine, increasing alertness and helping one think clearly. Particularly important are foods high in protein, vitamin D, omega fatty acids, B vitamins, carbohydrates and zinc. It is important to consult with a health care professional for an individualized supplementation of vitamins and minerals after a brain injury. Eating a healthy diet is beneficial because there are disruptions in brain chemicals which impact daily brain functioning such as cloudy thinking or problems with memory. It is important to consume the right amount of nutrients to improve these functions.

Healthy brain care is not just eating healthy and exercising. It involves healthy sleep hygiene, stress management and using memory compensatory skills that one may not have learned before their injury. After a brain injury most people expect to return to normal "just because the brain should." Most forget that before the injury the brain needed daily care to improve or maintain memory and attention. The brain carries a ton of information throughout the day and it also sheds a lot of information that we don't need to carry with us. After an injury, most people will focus on the information the brain is shedding versus the information it is holding onto. The physicians, family and injured become more concerned with the physical trauma and sometimes overlook what has occurred in the brain. We also have an issue with being unable to comprehend the injury since it is not visibly noticed. We fail to understand the emotional, cognitive, behavioral problems and/or frustration.

Besides the obvious functions that our brain is responsible for (i.e. heart rate, sleep control, lung functioning and the proper functioning of all other organs), the brain regulates other important skills. These important skills include: attention, memory, processing speed, problem solving, language abilities, emotions, thoughts and behaviors. The following paragraphs will explain in detail how these skills apply to our daily functioning.

Attention skills are needed on a daily basis. We need to be able to focus on information in our environment in order to understand and manipulate the information. Attention skills help maintain our arousal and alertness. Attention skills fluctuate throughout the day depending on our biological rhythms. For example, attention skills start to decrease after lunch and mental fatigue usually sets in. Our attention skills set the groundwork for remembering information which allows the brain to undergo more complicated thinking processes. We need attention to keep us alert, aroused and to make quick decisions throughout the day. When driving we make split second decisions based on how alert we are and how our brain filed our past experiences and quick retrieval thereof. We react without conscious effort.

Memory is a complicated process for the brain. It entails attending to information, encoding the information, organizing, storing and then retrieving the information when needed. There are different types of memory: auditory memory, visual memory, working memory, declarative memory, procedural or automatic memory and semantic memory. The brain uses all these memories on a daily basis. For example, the brain has the task to remember what has to be completed at work or at home, or remembering a special event such as a birthday, remembering how to drive a car or how to get to the grocery store.

Processing information is another important aspect of brain functioning. This involves our reaction time or our speed of thoughts. This plays a role with other functions including attention, memory, organizing, planning and executive functions. Processing information helps us take in and consolidate information.

The brain functioning referred to as the manager or executive director of all brain components is the executive functioning. The executive functions involve the process of how we do things. This includes planning, organizing, controlling, directing, setting goals, initiating activities, making sense out of information, decision making and problem solving. We do all of these skills on a daily basis at home, at work and while engaging in social activities.

Our language, sensory awareness and perceptual skills are also vital components needed to understand our world. Language involves comprehending and expressing words. Language is controlled from the left side of our brain. The sensory and perceptual skills include understanding information from our senses (i.e. hearing, vision, sound and touch) are found on the upper portion of the brain.

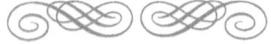

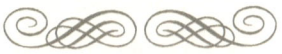

CHAPTER 3

The Brain in Emergency Situations

Stress impacts emotional, behavioral and physical reactions. There are certain stressors that are normal and healthy. It is the unhealthy stressors that negatively impact the brain, the emotions, behaviors and physical functioning. Let us take a look at how our brain reacts to stress especially in emergency situations or trauma. This research started back in the early 1950's by a scientist named Hans Seyle.

There are biological changes that occur when reacting to stress. Hans Seyle referred to this as a General Adaption Syndrome. There are three levels to this: an alarm reaction, a resistance response and exhaustion. Basically, these three levels entail biological changes.

During the alarm reaction, the nervous system becomes activated, also known as fight or flight. The unconscious brain informs the body to be on guard, therefore, the heart rate increases, breathing increases and skin reactions occur. This happens without us having to think; our brain merely reacts.

Resistance will occur if the stressor continues. Eventually, if the stressor continues over a longer period of time, the pituitary gland releases too much of an adrenocorticotrophic hormone. This hormone is comparable to a cleanup program that we use on our computers to improve the hard drive operation. However, too much release of this hormone over time will negatively wreak havoc on the brain and body. This means that if too much of this hormone is released it lowers immune responses and increases susceptibility to disease. This significantly reduces the ability to heal after a brain injury.

The last level, called exhaustion, can lead to detrimental consequences, including death. The body's defenses fail; the brain's functions shut down. In most cases, after a brain injury, the body is under a constant state of stress, as the brain is trying to heal. When one is constantly worried or concerned about what they are not able to do since their brain injury, the adrenocorticotrophic hormone level increases. This leads to a vicious stress response cycle.

When the brain reacts to an emergency situation (i.e. trauma, fear), emotions intensify. An emotion is different than a thought. An emotion is a feeling that is either pleasant or unpleasant. After a brain injury, which most likely was an emergency situation, the feelings tend to be unpleasant resulting in a stress response. During an emergency response, the feelings are usually fear. When we experience fear, adrenaline increases. This is due to the norephinerine and epheniprine increase in the brain. These brain transmitters make us more numb to any physical responses (i.e. we have heard stories about individuals lifting outrageous weighted objects if a loved one is trapped under said object). After the emergency response, the daily emotion is a post traumatic anxiety response. Other post-injury emotions that occur are frustration, irritability, hopelessness, depression and anxiety. It is usually the fear that sparks most of these trajectories of emotions. Fear can prevent the brain from healing in an optimum manner. This too can become a vicious cycle.

There are many different theories about how our brains operate when presented with fear. Some theorists suggest we think, then feel, then react. Other theorists propose that we react physically, then have the feelings and the thoughts follow. People are all unique and each of us have our own way to react to events. The brain and the heart operate together to create emotions. The meaningful traumatic emotional reactions also create memories which are stored in particular areas in the brain. Therefore, the brain regulates and holds onto the traumatic memories.

The brain operates our memory system. This memory system functions differently during an emergency situation when compared to our day-to-day memory functioning. During a trauma the brain will archive particular pieces of information almost like a camera taking snapshot pictures. When this information is archived it tends to be forgotten. A memory is how we retrieve and hold onto past information, events or experiences. The part of the brain, called the hippocampus, helps store and remember information. It operates like an online library, for example, keeping track of information about where and when events occurred.

Unfortunately, when the brain is faced with fear or trauma, the hippocampus doesn't function very well. Memories may not be tracked with information related to time or place and sometimes the information gets stored in the wrong area. Then, when information is recalled about the fear or trauma, it will feel like it is re-occurring again.

The memory process can be complicated to understand. It entails many interconnected neural networks which hold onto and retrieve information. There is also a memory for sensory information. During a trauma, many sensory memories are stored, but the trauma can also block the memory system. This is similar to post traumatic stress symptoms. This block creates difficulty connecting information, categorizing information, recalling thoughts and experiences. When information cannot be recalled, it makes it much more difficult to learn new ideas or retrieve old ones. As a result the injured person cultivates frustration or anger. It can also do the reverse: playing one event over and over; recycling information; or focusing on emotional memories, inconsistencies or the trauma itself.

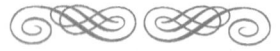

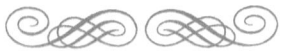

CHAPTER 4

The Injured Brain

There are many different types of brain injuries and they are classified as mild, moderate and severe. Brain injuries can occur from hitting one's head, a puncture into the brain, concussions, strokes, aneurysms and bleeds, just to name a few. When the brain is injured, depending on the severity of the injury, the injuries do not always show up on a CT (scan or x-Ray of the brain) or MRI (magnetic resonance image of the brain tissue). Often even severe injuries cannot be identified using these tests. That is why it is sometimes called the invisible injury. Brain injury symptoms vary among individuals because every brain is unique, except for the basic brain functioning. Imagine our brains similar to the largest library in the world and then one day a major earthquake happens. As you may be thinking, a lot of information probably got shifted around, buried, stuck somewhere, damaged or just lost. However, a year after the earthquake the library is rebuilt with more unique areas, new information and different access to the information. The "different access" can be a quick explanation of neuroplasticity-rebuilding new pathways in the brain. It is not exactly the way it was before, similar to our brain's functioning while recovering from an injury.

Brain injuries can also be categorized into direct and indirect injuries, which helps us understand how the brain reacts. A direct injury involves nerve fibers and axons that shred and tear, bruising from hitting the inside of the skull, bleeding or from a blood clot that puts pressure on the brain. Indirect injury involves anything related to swelling, infections, a slow bleed, anoxia or exposure to chemicals.

There are two important measures used to indicate the severity of the brain injury: 1) the loss of consciousness and 2) the level of post traumatic amnesia. The loss of consciousness is measured by one's response to their environment and the Glasgow coma scale which measures the depth of the coma or consciousness. The lower the score, the more severe the brain injury. For example, if one is not responding at all, they are most likely in a coma state. There are eight known levels of coma ranging from complete unresponsiveness, delayed responses, confused agitation, impaired judgment and decreased abilities to reason.

Many unusual and odd sensations, emotional, behavioral and neurological symptoms occur after a brain injury. This can happen after a mild, moderate or severe traumatic brain injury or concussion. Most doctors or emergency physicians only inform patients of the obvious symptoms of brain injury including: nausea, headache and sleepiness.

There are many common symptoms after a brain injury. They can be categorized into: emotional, cognitive, behavioral, physical and neurological. Some common symptoms individuals have after a brain injury are:

- ☐ brain feeling foggy
- ☐ feeling like one is in someone else's body learning everything new
- ☐ feeling like someone is constantly pulling on their brain
- ☐ avoiding family and friends because the injured feels inadequate due to thoughts failing to process

The emotional symptoms can vary:

- ☐ anxiety
- ☐ depression
- ☐ apathy (i.e. the lack of emotional responses, flat affect, lack of motivation)
- ☐ frequent unexplained crying
- ☐ uncontrollable laughter
- ☐ difficulty crying
- ☐ mood swings
- ☐ irritability
- ☐ lower frustration tolerance
- ☐ short fused
- ☐ difficulty controlling anger

The cognitive symptoms can vary:

- ☐ short and long term memory problems
- ☐ easily forgetting daily plans or routines
- ☐ easily distracted
- ☐ getting stuck on words
- ☐ problems with organizing, planning and problem solving
- ☐ difficulties understanding complex information when reading or listening to others
- ☐ poor or slow processing speed
- ☐ depth perception such as visuo-spatial problems
- ☐ lack of insight with the deficits
- ☐ tuning out without realizing it

Various behavioral symptoms:

- ☐ poor social skills
- ☐ impulsivity with decision making
- ☐ no social filter (e.g. speak ones thoughts without considering the consequences)
- ☐ withdrawal

Physical and neurological symptoms include, but not limited to:

- ☐ increase or decrease in sleep
- ☐ increase or decrease in appetite
- ☐ headaches
- ☐ fatigue

- ☐ changes in vision
- ☐ ringing in the ears
- ☐ sensitivity to noise (machines, fans, lawnmowers)
- ☐ sensory loss such as lack of smell or taste
- ☐ balance problems
- ☐ poor motor coordination
- ☐ increase or decrease in sexual desires or appetite
- ☐ reduced mobility in moving one's body
- ☐ seizures
- ☐ sensitivity to light, television or computer screens
- ☐ nausea brought on by light or sound

Although this list appears significant, each individual will experience and relate to an injury differently. This list is far from complete.

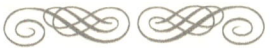

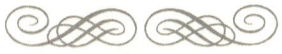

CHAPTER 5

How The Brain Heals

How long does it take the brain to heal? This is a great and complex question. An easy answer from treating professionals will be "after three to six months you are as good as you will be, there is no more healing to be done and you will never be 100%." I have heard this comment from patients often, usually when their treating professionals don't know how to work with them any further or they can't. Imagine the brain similar to a very intelligent computer that can rewire itself without having a virus. Currently, there is a lot of updated research to show that the brain will continue to heal or rewire itself for many years after an injury (neuroplasticity). The largest roadblock for many individuals is how they compare their current brain activity after their injury to their old functioning brain. Imagine the brain as a computer with new programs and then it crashes. It is rebuilt with newer software because the old software is outdated but it may have lost some of the old programs.

There are other unusual symptoms that occur after brain injuries in which there is no documented, quantitative research. These symptoms have been reported and demonstrated by patients:

- heightened senses including but not limited to hearing or vision
- increase in feelings, smell or taste

Some individuals become more intuitive, have iconic hearing, premonitions or become more creative. Unfortunately, there has been no documented research to prove to our society these findings. If one shares these symptoms they are perceived as having a thought disorder similar to schizophrenia.

However, there is documented research that demonstrates how the brain physiologically heals itself. In 1914, Von Monahow established that the non-injured parts of the brain physiologically connect with the injured areas of the brain, which helped improve daily functioning. This process can take a very long time. For example, the timeframe for healing after a brain injury depends on the severity of the injury and the stress level of the individual as well as the physical components (sleep, diet, exercise) previously discussed. In a moderate to severe injury, the brain can take 2 to 3 years to continue healing. The most noticeable healing occurs within the first 6 months after the injury. If the injury is mild, the recovery timeframe and rates are faster. In a mild injury, the cognitive, emotional and behavioral functioning can improve up to 90% within 12 months. There is newer research that demonstrates how recovery depends on the severity of the brain injury (Smith et al., 2013). If the injury is more serious the axons actually break instead of stretching or tearing. If the axon breaks, it releases too much protein and chemicals which can further damage nearby axons and dendrites. Even though the broken axon doesn't grow back, it will find and create new axons to connect to, another example of neuroplasticity.

From a biological perspective, there is evidence that supports learning and experiences creating physical changes in the brain. This also applies to brain injuries. There are neurological changes that occur within the actual neurons. Neurons have axons, synapsis and dendrites that sprout and connect to other ones in the brain. If a neuron is damaged it will sprout and connect using the axons, synapsis and dendrites to a neuron that is not damaged. This process is called neuroplasticity, which is evidenced in normal learning and the healing of a brain injury. In 1949, a renowned scientist, Donald Hebb, found that synaptic connections occur when neurons are activated at the same time. In sum, neurons that "fire together, wire together." Most people assume that any type of rehabilitation involves just changing a behavior to compensate, however, it needs to be perceived as a physiological/biological change as well.

There will be times of relapse. If the brain injured person is under an unusual amount of stress, hasn't slept well or their diet is off, they may experience the return of symptoms. Rather than be alarmed, realize correcting the stress overload or the other dynamics will aid in a return to better health and or thinking.

Allow the time you need to rest, recuperate and revive instead of becoming overwhelmed. This technique works for any injury or trauma.

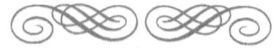

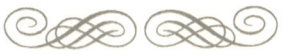

CHAPTER 6

The Use of Tools and Compensatory Skills to Heal

There are different treatment approaches that are beneficial to healing after a brain injury. The best approach is to address the bio-psycho-social aspects. This means not just addressing the brain functioning, but also the emotional, behavioral, physical, social and spiritual aspects. There is no "cookie cutter quick fix" therapy to address all these areas, which most individuals in our society try to find. There are many different approaches. Finding the best fit is the most important. In this chapter we will discuss the importance of addressing the cognitive, emotional and behavioral aspects which need to be combined with the proper nutrition, restorative sleep, exercise, mental relaxation and learning to manage stress in a healthy manner. All of these aforementioned factors will foster a healthy recovery. The following paragraphs will briefly discuss psychotherapy, cognitive rehabilitation, biofeedback and hypnosis.

Drugs impede the healing process. Rest promotes healing. Any activity that aids in sorting and organizing (such as the game of solitaire) or learning anything new (including knitting or a different language) also promotes healing.

Psychotherapy is one treatment modality that can address the emotional and behavioral symptoms that follow after a brain injury. Talking to a professional who has knowledge about brain injuries and posttraumatic stress disorder will be more beneficial than a professional who does not have familiarity. There are many different types of professionals who can provide psychotherapy. There are many different styles and strategies that treating professionals use. It is important to inquire about their style at the onset of treatment. According to recent research, cognitive behavioral therapy is the most effective in the shortest time frame. Managed health care and personal injury protection insurance companies only provide short term authorizations.

Cognitive behavioral therapy was developed by Aaron Beck and involves the work of many other renowned cognitive behavioral theorists including Beck, Lazarus, Ellis and Meichenbaum. The purpose of cognitive behavioral therapy is to understand one's thoughts and how thoughts apply to one's behaviors and emotions. Residual symptoms from a brain injury often lead to the individual's perceiving themselves, their current life experiences and the future as negative or hopeless. They believe their issues are permanent problems. Understanding behaviors and beliefs that are underlying most thoughts can improve one's outlook on life. When quality of life is altered due to a brain injury there are distorted beliefs that can prevent healthy healing. In psychotherapy these distorted beliefs can be brought to one's awareness. The psychotherapist can guide one in changing the beliefs to reflect healthier perceptions. Changing one's beliefs and thoughts can also be accomplished with hypnosis, which will be discussed in more detail in chapter 7.

Another treatment modality is cognitive rehabilitation. Cognitive rehabilitation targets relearning or new learning of cognitive skills that have been altered due to damage to brain cells or changes in brain chemistry. It is similar to engaging in physical therapy for an injured muscle or ligament. Cognitive rehabilitation can be a lengthy process with a cognitive therapist, which is different than a therapist who performs cognitive behavioral therapy. The rehabilitation can range from 6 to 24 months. Changes may be noticeable after 3 to 6 months from the time one starts treatment. Cognitive Rehabilitation usually includes a clinical interview and diagnostic evaluation. The diagnostic evaluation is called a neuropsychological examination which measures the brains functioning with regards to memory, attention, concentration, focusing, speech production, organizing, planning, visual motor skills, processing speed and achievement functioning. After the neuropsychological testing is completed, cognitive rehabilitation may be recommended to address the dysfunctional areas of the brain. The therapy needs to be tailored to the individual to help the injured party learn skills and strategies. The components of cognitive rehabilitation involve education about the difficulty of the brain's functioning, direct cognitive exercises such as memory and attention tasks, using computer programs or workbooks, learning compensatory skills and learning how to apply these skills to everyday life.

Over the years in providing treatment with my patients I have found significant objective improvements pre and post treatment. The treatments included: psychotherapy, pre and post neuropsychological testing, cognitive rehabilitation therapy and biofeedback. The archival data from 20 patients who received intensive treatment for 9-12 months documents the significant positive changes in their memory, attention and language deficits. The scores alone from the neuropsychological testing measuring memory and language functioning increased from 12-20 points. This is a significant increase based on the psychological statistics. These improvements may have been more impressive if those individuals also utilized a hypnosis component to their intensive treatment.

Biofeedback is another strategy of treatment which involves learning how to relax involuntary body responses such as breathing and heart rate. It is conducted by a biofeedback technician. There are many types of biofeedback. However, the main function is to teach self-control with thoughts while actually seeing the breathing and heart rate on a computer screen or monitor. This is usually done by monitoring skin temperature, heart rate, blood pressure, brain waves and other body functions.

Basic behavioral relaxation started in the early 1920's by Edmund Jacobson, a medical doctor from Chicago who coined the term progressive muscle relaxation. He explained that the body cannot be relaxed and anxious simultaneously. Jacobson explained how our thoughts influence muscle tension. If one learns how to conduct deep muscle relaxation, it will reduce physiological responses to anxiety, thus becoming a habit of responding to stressors. Progressive muscle relaxation involves tensing and then relaxing each muscle within the body.

There is another type of muscle relaxation called passive relaxation. Passive relaxation involves the same procedures as progressive muscle relaxation except there is no tensing and releasing involved. The relaxation involves providing a cue to imagine relaxing each muscle while engaging in deep breathing.

A very important component to these relaxation methods is the ability to use guided imagery. One form of guided imagery entails focus and concentration on each muscle as the body is relaxing. Stress can be reduced by the power of thinking and imagination. In 1882, a French pharmacist, Emile Coue, believed that the power of imagination is more powerful than one's will. He believed thoughts play a powerful role in our physical symptoms. For example, if one had worried thoughts it would make our body tense, thus increasing anxiety. Coue also suggested getting into a relaxed position and implanting the healthy ideas and thoughts to one's emotions and behaviors. He was famous for his line of "Every day in every way, I am getting better and better." He believed that he could teach people self-healing which resulted in physical changes. Therefore, some modern forms of hypnosis are based on his doctrine. Unfortunately, it took at least half of a century to be accepted into the medical field. Hypnosis will be discussed in more detail in chapter 7.

Coue's idea of implanting healthy thoughts was later followed up by Martin Seligman, who named the concept as Positive Psychology in 1998, but the idea was actually originated by Abraham Maslow in 1954. Seligman sparked the empirical beginning of how positive thoughts changed our emotions. Since this time there has been much focus on positive psychology and mindfulness in the healing fields and how it improves our emotional and physical healing. We need to understand that our thoughts are influenced by ingrained belief systems. These belief systems are shaped and developed from the time we arrive in this world. These influences stem from parents, teachers, friends, school, work and many other social influences including movies, television and other media. Belief systems influence how we perceive our world, our families and overall life. Belief systems also influence our values in relationships, finances, work ethic, education, religion, spiritualness, how we managed unpleasant events and feelings and about how we help ourselves when we become injured or sick.

Research has found that as people grow older they increase their focus on positive events and happier feelings. In MRI's it was found that individuals who are older and concentrate on joy and happiness had stronger activity showing in their amygdala and the prefrontal cortex within the brain. The amygdala regulates emotions as the prefrontal cortex regulates daily decision making. In 2013, Mara Mather and her colleagues found that there is greater activity in brain circuits linking the amygdala when shown happy and positive faces within older individuals as compared to younger people.

Changing thoughts to reflect positive thoughts can be done with cognitive behavioral therapy and hypnosis. Hypnosis will also reinforce the change. The goal is to change the negative style of thoughts to reflect more positive thoughts and emotions. In turn this will lead to positive changes about how we think about ourselves, about other people and about our future in regards to injuries as well as our overall health.

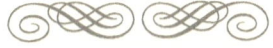

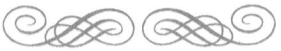

CHAPTER 7

How to Revitalize and Rewire the Brain

Hypnosis is a form of creative visualization or guided imagery. They all work in the same part of the brain, that which uses imagination and creativity. Hypnosis normally consists of a skilled, trained hypnotist helping a client enter a relaxed state to produce a result such as stress reduction or a behavioral change. The hypnotist taps into the part of the brain that we use when we daydream, relax or meditate.

There are many different levels of hypnosis and an individual will only go to the level they are comfortable with. Whether one is using self-hypnosis or being guided by a therapist or hypnotist, the individual will go to the place they feel safe. Even in somnambulism, a state similar to sleep, one must feel comfortable and safe or it is doubtful the state can be reached. In the case of hypnosis it is the state of ultra depth and may be an effective manner for change to occur. In my experience individuals need or like to know and be aware of self-discovery and change so the lighter states of hypnosis work well.

I have found in my practice when a client goes into a somnambulistic state, they are very relaxed but have no memory of the session. They don't understand what took place. That often leads to confusion. In a session a client may drift in and out of deeper states of consciousness. It has been apparent that my clients appreciate the guidance and retain an awareness of the process that is relaxing and rejuvenating.

A Harvard research study demonstrated that hypnosis actually builds brain cells (Holzel et al. 2011). A research team at Massachusetts General Hospital, led by Harvard affiliated researchers, concluded that hypnosis increases gray matter and builds brain cells in the brain. These physiological changes were found with using magnetic imaging (MRI). The participants spent eight weeks engaging in a mindful meditation program and listened to guided mediation 27 minutes daily. The MRI's were conducted two weeks before they began the study and then at the end of the eight weeks. They also utilized a control group who had MRI's and did not engage in the mindful meditation. The results showed that gray matter (that part of the brain that we don't know how it is used but we do know it is the part that can be used to redevelop cognitive aspects of the brain) decreased in the amygdala and the gray matter increased in the hippocampus. Basically, the research found with meditation the brain builds brain cells and increases gray matter in the areas of the brain that control learning, memory, self-awareness, introspection and compassion. In other words, meditation helps heal brain functioning.

Hypnosis and meditation can produce similar results but have different intentions. They both provide deep, meaningful experiences that will change over time while gaining self-knowledge. There are important aspects of hypnosis and meditation: purpose and motivation, style and technique, assessment of suggestibility and actual suggestions for future behaviors. Both cause relaxation, contentment and serenity. Sessions can be conducted individually or with groups. While in the state of hypnosis or meditation, time becomes distorted and muscles release tension. After a session most individuals report a good night's sleep. Individuals also report a wide range of thoughts, feelings and dreams.

There are differences between hypnosis and meditation. Frequently, meditation is used for stress reduction, improving sleep, taking a mental break, relaxation or developing insights. Hypnosis is different in terms of motivation. Most people will seek out hypnosis for smoking cessation, health benefits, stress reduction, weight reduction and to improve confidence. The intention of hypnosis is to open the subconscious mind to suggestions. During hypnosis, individuals are awake but in a state of detachment. They suspend critical thinking or self-criticism and permit their creative genius to explore and activate.

Meditation and hypnosis both use an infinite number of suggestions. With hypnosis, the suggestions are fitted to the individual's needs to permit the conscious mind to allow a trance-like state. In a hypnosis group, the hypnotist will provide a variety of suggestions in order to appeal to each individual's learning style. Techniques used for hypnosis include deepeners, ego strengthening and anchoring.

In the intake or interview, the hypnotist determines the individual's learning method such as visual, kinesthetic or auditory. All types are good. None is better than any other. Both hypnosis and meditation are very powerful for personal transformation, improvement and development.

Meditation can be relaxing and clearing. Some forms of meditation such as transcendental meditation focus on a mantra and clearing the mind of all thought. With practice and time, the individual becomes open to insights. Other forms of meditation may focus on a spiritual awareness.

Guided visualization is a method of using a script, similar to hypnosis, to tap into the creative areas of the brain promoting awareness. A simple guided visualization would be to imagine your muscles relaxing and remembering perfect health.

Hypnosis utilizes relaxation techniques to assist the individual. Progressive relaxation suggests the muscles tighten then relax beginning with either the toes or head and slowly progressing throughout the body until complete relaxation occurs. There are suggestibility tests such as holding a brick or weight in one hand and a balloon in the other. Most hypnotists use scripts.

A positive attitude and positive affirmations are needed in order for hypnosis to work. If one doesn't believe it will work, it will not. If an individual can return to a time in their life when they had a healthy affirmation or a positive attitude, they will be able to relax and remember it. Once an individual believes the healthy affirmation or positive attitude, it can be re-created and then healing will occur with feeling. Our heart holds our emotions and our emotions work with our brains. If it is true that our heart holds our emotions, then during hypnosis we can transport that feeling to the brain.

Stress negatively impacts the brains functioning and the ability to meditate or use hypnosis effectively. When one is under stress there usually is a specific focus on the stressor. When this happens one may overlook something wonderful that's creative. If the creative energy becomes negated, an individual will become too focused on the stressor and possibly be unable to meditate. When one is stressed, the brain is on overload which prevents learning, refocusing or absorbing anything. Stress is usually connected to a message from old beliefs passed on from parents, teachers or mentors that perfection is expected and if one fails they are not good enough. However, our old beliefs forget to mention that we are perfect the way we are. We are human and can understand or learn from our mistakes. Being intelligent doesn't mean we know anything. It only means we can learn anything we desire to learn. We can be successful in any field or endeavor we choose, even with a brain injury.

When our brains are in a stress mode, there are physiological changes that are occurring. When we are confronted with a stressor, our brains send a signal to our bodies to increase heart rate, increase breathing, redistribute our blood flow in our bodies, dilate the pupils and then too many brain chemicals may be released. This is a complicated system that occurs but just one stressor will set off the stress cycle. When one is under constant stress, the part of the brain, the hypothalamus, continues to be activated. The glucocorticoid hormone allows one to remain in the fight against the stressor, which is used as the continued energy to cope. Compare these hormones to a tune up in an engine. When an engine is tuned up it needs less work or less gas. However, with our bodies the continued release of hormones make us use more energy and less food. Overtime, constant glucocorticoid releasing can be detrimental to the brain, as well as the body. Frequently, the brain issue is overlooked.

How Our Brain Interprets Reality

Our brains are magnificent creatures. Each one of us has a different and special way to view reality. No way is better than any other. None are wrong or incompatible with reality. I do a lot of work with having my client go to the initial sensitizing event. That's when the person first dealt with the situation or has imprinted a belief or idea about the problem. Most often, my client will go to a childhood event. Sometimes the client is remembering what I call genetic encoding. Genetic encoding is remembering something in the family lineage that occurred to a biological distant relative or someone adopted into the family or entered the family through marriage. I have a way to remove the pattern the client is holding as their own. But that's not where I'm going now. I'm about to tell you a story of my mother's experience with her initial event, which explains how hypnosis can rewire our thoughts and beliefs.

Twenty five years ago I had the pleasure of having a dog and a cat. They were lovable creatures. When I traveled or went to conferences I had to place them in what I referred to as their vacation location. All went well until Titan, my beloved dog, came home with a cough. I vowed they would be cared for at home. Everyone I knew either worked away from home or was fearful of Titan. My mother said if I helped her overcome her fear, she would consider pet sitting. Titan was a mixed Labrador.

So we had a session. Not utilizing my psychic abilities in the healing environment unless my client gave me permission to do so, I assumed El, my mother, had issues with her older brother's dog. I had heard stories about her childhood and how she wouldn't enter the yard if the dog was loose. After El was relaxed enough to allow her creative mind to remove unnecessary filters, she permitted her imagination to wander. That's how hypnosis works. We allow the process to take place. She traveled through time back to her childhood, then, suddenly, she was looking down on trees that had red fruit. As I asked her questions she discovered she was a little boy about 5 or 6 or 7 somewhere in Europe. She/he had wandered away from home into the orchard to play. She/he lost all track of time. An animal began to stalk the child. Becoming fearful, she/he climbed up one of the trees. It became cold. The wolf at the base of the tree wasn't leaving. The animal of prey sat patiently waiting for nightfall. The child's parents looked for the little one but in the wrong directions. As it got colder, the child fell asleep, lost her/his footing and fell to the ground. The hungry predator...... you can imagine the outcome. One would think El should remain fearful through all time. But I knew how to resolve the fears. I walked her/him through the death scenario, tailored a forgiveness exercise and brought El back to the consciousness of the room.

Her face was so peaceful. She was smiling. She told me how happy she felt and she understood something about forgiveness that I had been trying to explain for years. She got it!! Then she asked where Titan was. I brought him into the room and she playfully petted and talked to him. After that she brought him toys and treats. This was a woman who didn't even want to see Titan before this experience. When she finally pet sat and had to go back home, she called to "talk" to Titan. Does it matter if her experience was real or imagined? Who cares! It helped her deal with a fear she harbored all her life.

Another experience El had with past life exploration dealt with being a pirate. Again, that's not where I thought we were going. We were dealing with determining the reason she had issues with one of her sisters. Within the experience, El found her sister betrayed her. Other members of the crew found out and threw the culprit overboard via "walking the plank." El wasn't sure if there was actually a plank but she was very happy the rest of her pirate com-padres supported her. She was the captain! El liked to be boss in anything she could in our present time line! I had El look around and find other pirates she might know in the present time. To her amazement and surprise, she saw her real life sister-in-law in the eagle's nest. El didn't have a vast vocabulary so she was describing it as "you know, that big seat up where the sails are. That place you can sit at to see what's up ahead." That's when, as a Hypnocounselor, one knows the client is telling the truth. She found me on that ship, also. I was a girl about 12 years old and not hers. She wasn't sure how I got there but I had beautiful dresses they confiscated from ships traveling from Paris. There were others she identified with the present.

When I inquired how she got her command, she was vague. Not that she didn't know, she just didn't want to say. And what about the ship itself? It took many, many questions for her to finally say, "We took it" being very embarrassed that I wouldn't let it go until she admitted her crime.

And where did you live or set up your port? The Caribbean. No wonder she liked cruising to those islands in this lifetime! And what was it like? It seems they had a good life hiding their loot, playing with some of it, trading it, until they had to fight with others who discovered their lair. But that's not what put her down in that lifetime. Drinking, singing and all the things one may think a pirate would do were on her list. "And what

41

happened that your life ended?" I inquired. "Well, we hit a really bad storm and we all went down together," she replied. "Was that fearful?" "Not at all." Drowning wasn't even an issue in this lifetime. She felt she had a wonderful life, was respected, had authority, was loved and enjoyed the life.

The real bonus was when she returned to this reality. Again, so very happy. The first comment and what she told many for years to come was "that was better than any movie." It was about the same time <u>Pirates of The Caribbean </u>came out so I purchased it for her. She said it was good but her experience was better. That's when I knew it was real for her. The additional benefit was that the issues she had with that sister no longer mattered to her.

This story about my mother demonstrates how old beliefs negatively impact current functioning, possibly preventing healthy healing. It clearly shows that hypnosis has the ability to change those old beliefs to reflect healthier and more functional beliefs.

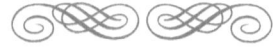

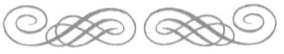

CHAPTER 8

How to Use your Brain to Promote Healing

Most professionals that treat individuals with brain injuries inform their patients of permanent outcomes as they begin treatment. For example, some commonly verbalized outcomes by professionals have been: "your injuries are permanent," "your brain is damaged," "accept the permanent changes," "accept this new behavior as your new normal,", and "don't expect your brain to improve after 6 months." However, as we discussed in chapter 5 regarding neuroplasticity, we do know the brain is amazing in healing on a physiological level, without any tools or skills. In this chapter the use of guided tools and skills, particularly with the use of hypnosis, will be discussed in conjunction with neuroplasticity abilities. Qualitative examples that revealed scientific evidence will be supplied as well.

Engaging in Functional Hypnosis, also referred to as Clinical Hypnosis, Hypnocounseling or Hypnotherapy, is not a replacement for traditional medical or mental health treatment and should not be used as such. Hypnosis is not a replacement for a primary physician's care nor is it to be used for, or is it a replacement of any medications, diagnosis or treatment by a licensed medical doctor. The success of hypnosis depends greatly on one's ability and desire to affect and believe in change. The results depend greatly on one's participation and follow through. Although hypnosis can be very effective and has a high success rate, there is no guarantee since one's personal success depends on the intent, follow up with exercises and visualizations that hypnosis offers and commitment to the program. Hypnosis does not magically make issues disappear. It only works for those who are willing to the take responsibility of healing. If one is willing to believe in it, understand it and take responsibility, it is a wonderful tool promoting our bodies to heal.

Secondary gain

One of the problems that we all run into is the effect or the interaction with our client with secondary gain. Secondary gain is the benefit one has in remaining ill. That may sound strange but it is an actual effect. If someone suffered or sustained an injury due to a trauma involving a case of liability there is a possibility of financial gain. Another type of secondary gain could be the attention and the support the injured party is receiving from others. In the short run, holding off becoming stronger or recovering may not be an issue. The problem becomes apparent when the injured party has learned coping skills that work for them that would maintain a low level of recovery. There could come a time when the new pattern of behavior overrides the benefit of healing. Rather than implying the injured party wants to maintain their injured brain and avoid becoming well, we are merely stating that subconsciously many of us have a benefit of secondary gain. To overcome the propensity of this situation one must realize the importance of working the muscle we are referring to as the brain. It is similar to atrophy of a bicep or tricep. Whatever we give attention to becomes enhanced.

There is a hierarchy of needs that must be met before one takes action to heal. If a person doesn't feel safe, nothing will overcome the fear. In 1943 Abraham Maslow, a renowned humanistic psychologist, coined the hierarchy of needs.

The hierarchy of needs includes:

1) Physiological needs—biological needs such as oxygen, food, water and warmth/coolness. These needs are the strongest because if they are deprived, one could die.
2) Safety and security needs—we all can feel these during emergencies or periods of trauma (shootings in schools, rioting, etc.). Children often fear the monster under their bed.
3) Love and belonging needs—The need to escape loneliness and alienation; the need to give and receive love, affection and a sense of belonging

4) Esteem needs—People need a stable, firmly based, high level of self-respect and respect from others in order to feel satisfied, self-confident and valuable.

5) Cognitive needs—The need to know and understand

6) Aesthetic needs—Symmetry, order and beauty

7) Self-actualization needs—To find self-fulfillment and realize one's potential

8) Transcendence needs—To help others find self-fulfillment and realize their potential

The use of hypnosis can improve the higher level of hierarchy of needs.

Besides the aforementioned, there is evidence that the use of hypnosis in the medical field creates positive results or changes. This evidence dates back to the early 1920's and 1930's by a well-known psychiatrist, Milton Erickson. He was also known as the greatest hypnotist in the 20th century. Milton Erikson published the first research in relation to using hypnosis in the medical field and demonstrated effective changes in health. It was published in the Journal of Abnormal and Social Psychology in 1932.

Milton Erikson's own use of hypnotism and recovery from polio was astonishing. When he was in high school he had been debilitated suddenly by polio, almost totally paralyzed. With the use of self-hypnosis, he recovered within 11 months and regained mobility and his speech. Then, he went off to medical school. He started the foundation for psychological healing through the use of hypnosis.

Milton Erikson's story was one of many documented physiological changes as a result of hypnosis. The following are our examples, from ourselves and from clients we treated: a client was diagnosed with breast cancer, and after 3 sessions of hypnosis the cancer was no longer found. Another client was diagnosed with colon cancer, and after several hypnosis sessions his surgery was cancelled due to the absence of cancer. In fact, he sent all of his family members to see Elaine for sessions because he felt we all could use a gentle attitude adjustment.

One of my healing journeys was when I was diagnosed with a thyroid colossal cyst, which is congenital, and consulted with an endocrinology surgeon who suggested that it be removed. I opted to wait, due to the concerns of vocal cord damage. After 6 months and twice a month hypnosis sessions the cyst dissolved and was no longer detectable. These are only a few of our client stories.

The following is Elaine's story: On March 31, 1977, March was leaving New Jersey with the roar of a lion. There was silence, then the sudden activity of the wind took over. Blustery gusts of wind prevailed. I was returning from lunch. As I walked across the parking lot I remember thinking whoever opened those doors must have them nicely secured. Not so. I approached the double doors during a moment of calm. Then, without warning, a huge gust of wind blew the door, unlocking it from its locked position and hurled it into my head. I was knocked away with my head bleeding and the inability to see. Something strange was happening. I couldn't think. I couldn't talk. I couldn't walk.

I vaguely remember being at a hospital then home. How I got there or home is a blank. Funny thing with head injuries-sometimes there is a moment of clarity and most of the time no recall at all. I attempted to go to work and was taken to Dr. O'Carroll, the workers compensation physician.

The forces of good were on my side. I was stuttering in phrases. I couldn't remember if I said something, just thought of it or if it was a new idea entirely. A wonderful orthopedic treating my mother didn't like the way I looked. He made sure I got to a Neurologist quickly. My actual diagnosis was contusions of the brain. I couldn't see out of my right eye for about 2 years. Hearing was impaired. My balance was off and I was walking into walls.

Talk about a misdiagnosis. The general practitioner thought I was depressed and placed me on a cocktail of things I didn't need. By the time the neurosurgeon saw the bottles of pills, I needed detox. He sent me to an interesting place to do that, Carrier Clinic. He ordered a lot of tests that were done at the local hospital. Within a week I was on the road to recovery and released myself against Carrier's advice. I asked what they were doing for me and got no response. I asked if I needed outside therapy and their reply was "no." I promised to see my neurosurgeon asap and did so.

The brain heals in its own way. My director at work understood the injury. We dealt with traumatic brain injuries. I was a Corporate Claims Consultant for tort (injury) claims. He confessed a few years later he didn't think I'd pull through as well as I did. Rather than giving me my usual assignments— which I was unable to comprehend at the time—he gave me busy work that a clerk could have accomplished. That rote work, making diagrams of the different legislation countrywide, actually helped my brain remember how to file information. I may have been doing this for 3 to 6 months. Slowly, I began to speak to people. I had been embarrassed with the confusion I was having so I kept away from everyone. My son, all of 9 years old, was my guiding light. He had to remember where I parked the car because I couldn't. He had to escort me through life because my balance was so unreliable and seeing thorough one eye was new to me.

Sounds were unbearable. If someone was running a lawn mower or a vacuum or even a washing machine, my head throbbed so badly I wanted to run away. And I did. I retreated to my room stuffed between pillows. Lights hurt. Color from the television gave me headaches.

During my recovery period I discovered a stack of aluminum trays about 3-4 feet high. I had no memory of eating. My parents were purchasing TV dinners I could make for myself. Why I saved the trays I'll never know. How I managed is a mystery to this day. I'm sure my parents helped but I was living alone with my child. How he got to school or led his life or if he was with me or my parents is a black hole in my memory.

So that was the first year. Slowly my activities began to normalize. I could go food shopping and get home. I managed to go to work. I needed a lot more sleep than I ever did before. I liked sitting in dark rooms. If I didn't get enough rest I would have disabling headaches. That still occurs all these years later. I become a bit over concerned about sleep because I fear those headaches. Some are so intense I have been known to vomit. Not a pleasant experience.

It was about year 2 after the trauma that my work normalized. Peripheral vision issues still haunt me from time to time. If I'm overtired my mind isn't as clear as it should be. Balance can still be questionable. Strobe lights make me ill. Loud sounds have become bearable but only if they are of a short duration.

One of the things people suffering from trauma avoid talking about is the resentment or confusion that occurs due to the loss of time. I lost a year of my life. I have little or no memory of that time. I lied about my age by one year because I felt cheated. Because I looked "normal" not many people understood my limitations. When I'm in pain or discomfort I might also be confused. My expression appears to be one of anger or disappointment when in reality it's just me being uncomfortable or in pain.

There are many ways to recover. I play solitaire or free cell to make sure my thought patterns are in check. I meditate. I walk. I clean. None of these activities are for fun. I find myself doing them more when I'm distressed or unclear. In the early 1980's I attended Life Spring workshops which really helped. How? It was like EST but with love. Everyone accepted me as I was. It helped that they didn't know how active I had been before the injury. If I was really quiet they just thought that was who I was. I was born talking. Quiet is not something that comes naturally for me. There was an exercise in an advanced course of Life Spring in which one spoke about their limitation and how the course helped them overcome the problem. I remember thanking the group of about 20-30 people for accepting me as I was without criticism if I couldn't remember something or if I was slow to respond. It was amazing how they didn't know of my misfortune, discovered it and accepted it. That experience gave me permission to accept my limitations and go forward. It took the pressure off. It opened me up to accepting that I could heal in the time I needed and if others didn't understand, that was their issue, not mine.

Today I allow the injury to be a part of me. I know what happens if I don't get sufficient sleep. I can hear my words get jumbled if I'm on overload. I give myself permission to kick back and meditate or wash a floor or whatever it takes to gather my strength. If my balance gets "off" I still get panicked but I do something to relax and get my oars back into the water. I realize my limitations without the confusion and regret I once had. I can't ride a bike and found that out a few years after the accident. I can't ski any longer because the snow appears flat white and I can't judge the depth without shadows. Instead, I focus on what I can do. I can travel, I can read, I can visit with family and friends, I can laugh, I can enjoy a good program, most important of all—I can love...... and the list is unlimited.

These stories demonstrate that hypnosis can promote the brains ability to naturally heal the body. Hypnosis has been used for many centuries to reduce physical ailments and stress related chronic pain, headaches, and many other emotional and physical discomforts.

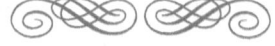

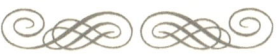

CHAPTER 9

The Brain: Emotions and Memory

We store memories in our body and in our brain. We feel things when we remember events that were on either side of the spectrum of happy or sad. It may be in our gut, our heart, our throat or anywhere else our body stored the event. When you remember a glorious day in your life, how do you remember it? Through NLP (NeuroLinguistic Programing) we learn that we feel, see, hear or use some other mechanism to recall events. When you close your eyes, what do you "see?" Is it black or gray? Are there colors? Are sparks of light perceived? We all process differently. No method is any better than any other.

So take a moment and "remember" something. How do you feel? Where in your body have you stored this memory? It can be "in your head" or you may have a feeling in your abdomen. Wherever it is, it is your choice or the way you learned to process. Close your eyes. Has your inner vision changed? As you remember the event has something changed in your body?

Now do the same with an unpleasant event. Remember it. Recall how you felt at the time. Notice how you are feeling as you remember it. Is there an unpleasantness somewhere? Where?

The Body Remembers

Our bodies store energy and memories. When you think of a pleasurable experience, your body recreates the event. It's similar to recalling the sourness of a lemon or the wind blowing through your hair as you ride a roller coaster. If the roller coaster was a fearful experience, you might feel the hairs on the back of your neck standing erect or your stomach doing a dive.

It has been my experience that not only do the charges of our present life scar our being but our past life experiences can also be remembered through these feelings. Does it matter if it was a past life, our childhood or something we perceived as real on TV? No. As long as we learn what the feelings are, how to release them and create a healthy life, we benefit. We never release those positive or loving feelings.

How do we locate what we've overlooked for so very long? How do we rationalize our illnesses or accidents? Could we really desire so deeply to improve or change that we ignore messages along the way until one finally gets our attention? Yes. That's the way we work. Our inner system only permits us to heal that which we are ready to work with. If we can't hear the message in a gentle manner, we keep having it delivered until we accept it. Pain, emotional or physical, is notifying us that something is wrong. If we don't experience some pain or discomfort, most of us would never change or grow.

The first step is to become quietly relaxed, noticing your breath, bringing yourself to a safe awareness of your body. As you become more relaxed you may notice sensations. But for the moment, concentrate on something that is bothering you. It doesn't have to be something traumatic. It could be a small issue. Ask your Higher Self, God, angels, guides, or whatever you believe in to help you find the answers you need.

As you relax, become aware of your heart rate. What else is going on in your body? Are you aware of any sensations? Heaviness, numbness, tingling, stiffness are all a part of the awareness. Is anything specifically hurting? Are emotions coming up? Any tears? Thank your body for cooperating with you.

What is your body attempting to tell you? Are you remembering an event? Is a particular body part guiding you to a realization? Is an old heartache blocking you from happiness? Are resentments keeping you stiff? Go into the part that is screaming for your attention. Lovingly, ask it what message it carries or what it wants you to know. When you've collected the information, thank the part again. Journal your findings. Allow yourself to gather more information over the next few days to complete the picture. Your inner guidance works when you're sleeping or awake. Allow the messages to arrive in a way that you can understand and accept them.

How does all of this relate to trauma? The event stopped you in your life path. Whatever was going on suddenly halted. You had to make changes in the way you perceived your future. I don't know anyone who, after a traumatic event, felt good about it. We are human. We feel guilt, regret, sorrow, you name it and it's there. Wallowing in self-pity or any negative state limits growth and healing. Becoming aware of the limitation opens one to acceptance and change. So your balance is off and you may never be able to wear high heels again. What if you can't throw a ball or ski again? Focus on what you can do. Explore new things you may never have thought of before. Live well in spite of your issues. Open your heart and mind to growth. If you can't read because you can't concentrate, DVR a program or get a book on CD or MP3 and play it in parts. So, if you must replay what you've already seen or heard, replay it. Eventually you will make progress. Some days it will be in leaps and bounds. Other days it will seem as if you are digressing. Rather than becoming angry, do what you can do. Eating and normal human activities are important.

And when you get over your self-incrimination, get busy helping others. Make a meal. Clean a bathroom. Do something no matter how insignificant you may think it is. It's progress. If you become depressed over your limits, you go deeper into the depths of sorrow. When you accept, practice, move forward, work within the constraints of your injury or pain, you heal much more rapidly. Try it for a day. Then go for a week. As you begin to notice small successes, more cascade into your life.

Many of our children and some of us have been told how brilliant we are. Intelligent, smart, gifted people are all around us. What we failed to realize was that we all have wonderful gifts. "They," those wonderful people who thought they were encouraging us, gave us a very mixed message. "They" didn't realize "they" were limiting us. What "they" either didn't know or had no way of communicating was that being intelligent simply means one has the ability to learn and do anything the individual desires to. It means we can practice and become specialists in any field. It doesn't mean we know everything; it merely means we have the capacity to learn anything. It's like success. How do you measure success? Are you using someone else's yardstick to determine your joy, success and abilities? Are you feeling less than because you couldn't accomplish something someone else had expectations of? And how do you feel about that? As one carries all of these negative emotions, we shut down our brain.

Our Reflection

The world surrounding us reflects our beliefs about ourselves. We attract experiences for our own growth. People enter our world to fulfill our request to learn, forgive, resolve and to love. They reflect anything we like or dislike in our lives or ourselves. When we "know" what another person is thinking, we are actually constructing a scenario based on our own experiences. When we decide what someone's expressions mean, we're interpreting their mannerisms based on what we recall from our early childhood. What did Mommy or Daddy look like when they hovered over our cribs when we cried or smiled? What postures did our teachers take when we failed or succeeded? We translate these early imprints to our bosses, friends and lovers. If they raised their voices or used harsh words, we're thrown back into earlier memories and react the way we did when we first heard them. Whether real or imagined, over the years we've accepted the negatives as true but often rejected the positive.

Changing the way we accept ourselves brings results. Depending on the way we change, these changes can eliminate some of the emotions that drain us. We no longer jump the gun when someone comments. We begin to comprehend that each individual has his/her personal road map of life. This map enables us to travel roads of experience. Without it, we feel lost. It is now time to rewrite and redraw the map.

Forgiveness sets us free. Instead of wallowing in the self-pity of the past, understand we do create our own experiences. It is not what is said or done that hurts us; it is our interpretation of the event. Realizing the other person's intent was not to poison our essence is an essential ingredient. People don't lie awake nights imagining ways to mistreat us. We just aren't that important. People in pain react defensively. They lash out with words or gestures. As we stop accepting the harsh behavior as our fault or problem, the negativity will lose its effect. As we walk away from turmoil, we take back our pride and perfection. We are all born perfect. We begin using a yardstick of performance as soon as we are weighed at birth. The measurements the infant becomes aware of instills security or lack thereof. Adults have no idea how judgmental they/we can be. We're taught a sense of perfection with our first breath. We learn no matter what we do, we can never achieve it! How can that be if we're born perfect? As we came to the planet, we forgot. We began permitting everyone to cut us down rather than lift us to greatness. So many authorities tell us to control our emotions. Why? Let's just stuff all our reactions and emotions deep inside until we experience depression, guilt, anxiety, loneliness and every other negative emotion. If we forgive ourselves for simply allowing these negative messages to hinder us, we take the first step. Doing exercises to forgive others for simply being human, realizing everyone has limitations, understanding what these experiences have taught us and realizing the society in which we live contribute to a new attitude.

Rather than controlling your emotions, feel them. Which parts help you survive? Which can you release? What do they teach you? Are you ready to remove the old walls of deception and allow love in? Can you now understand everyone is experiencing some type of pain? Does this comprehension allow you to become free? Will you now accept positive experiences? Forgiveness sets you free. Freedom permits you to control your life. Freedom opens new doors.

Now imagine how someone with a head injury may feel. Perhaps they feel as though they are always being judged. Are they living up to the expected progress? I'm certain they feel misunderstood. If they were once energetic and happy they may now be confused and depressed. Wouldn't you be? After having a life filled with hope and dreams of the future, one with a traumatic brain injury (or any other type of trauma) now needs to develop a new lifestyle with many limitations. If we can learn to slowly accept each hurdle and learn a new path, life can be a bit easier. Mounting expectations only create boundaries and walls. Accepting each triumph no matter how tiny allows us to take baby steps which lead us to a path of recovery. Stop expecting what was previously normal. Allow the injured time to heal to the best possible degree. When things are good, play or work. When times are difficult, rest or recuperate planning for tomorrow without regret.

As you remember how you store your memories, have you wondered if you can change the way you feel about the past event? Well, you can. Anything that is similar to love will always resonate as a positive, joyful memory. You have the ability to stop the past event that has been wearing you down and wearing you out from controlling your behaviors and beliefs. All you need to do is realize that the old memory is draining you. You are permitting a past event to steal your energy, your emotions, your future! There are many ways to reframe the old pattern, belief, issue or memory. Once you realize how it is affecting you in the present you can make a determination to release it.

Find your very best candle, the prettiest one with the most delectable fragrance. Turn down the lights and sit comfortably. As you light your candle stare into the flame and allow all of your thoughts to gently burn away. Let all of your troubles go up in smoke as you continue to stare into your luscious, lighted candle. Allow yourself to fly away or use your imagination as the flame flickers. Find yourself relaxing even more as you gently defocus your gaze. Do this from one to ten minutes to allow your brain to relax and retrain. As you become more and more relaxed, you will find that you heal at a rate that may be more rapid then when you were filled with stress or the variety of thoughts you couldn't turn off. You might even notice that as you are staring into the candle's flame your entire body relaxes and your breathing becomes slower or more comfortable. You might find that as you focus on your flame you tune out the negative energy of the world and you create a safe, sacred space.

This exercise is a form of meditation. It requires no thought. As you permit your thought patterns to ebb and flow you might even find harmony in your body. You have an opportunity to create a new reality for yourself; a reality of comfort, healing, tranquility. Enjoy your new found way of relaxation as you heal physically, mentally or emotionally. You decide.

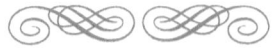

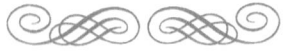

REFERENCES

1. Holzel, Carmody, Vangel, Congleton, Yerramsetti, Gard, & Lazar, 2011, 1,191. Psychiatry Research Neuroimaging. Mindfulness Practice Leads to Increases in Regional Brain Gray Matter Density.
2. Mather, Sakaki, & Nga, 2013, 8, 25. Cognitive Neuroscience. Amygdala Functional Connectivity with Medial Prefrontal Cortex at Rest Predicts Positivity Effect in Older Adults Memory.
3. Fuch, Bajjalien, Hoffman, & Greenough, 1983, 9, 54. Regional Brain 2-deoxyglucose
Uptake during performance of learned task. Society of Neuroscience Abstracts.
4. Smith, D. Et al. Nature Reviews of Neuorlogy, vol.9, 2013.

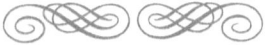

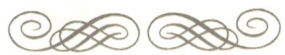

ABOUT THE AUTHORS

Sheryl Gallo is a licensed clinical psychologist/neuropsychologist specializing in diagnosis and treatment of neurocognitive disorders and brain injury. She received her doctorate of psychology from Philadelphia College of Osteopathic Medicine and holds two master's degrees in clinical and forensic psychology. She has a private practice in New Jersey.

Elaine Billy is a consultant and hypnocounselor specializing in communication, relationships, motivation and empowerment. Her credentials include holding a bachelor's degree of science in management with a minor in psychology from Rutgers University, being a neurolinguistic programming practitioner, being a certified clinical master hypnocounselor, being a certified master motivational specialist, and recipient of Order of Braid, one of the highest designations a hypnotist can achieve. After a lucrative career in the insurance industry, Elaine left her upper-management position to enter the field of healing modalities.

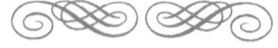